The Sugar Switch

The Powerful Key to Lose Weight,
Look Good and *Feel Great!*

Praise for The Sugar Switch

The Powerful Key to Lose Weight, Look Good and Feel Great!

"Cathy has written the perfect book for anyone that wants to flip The Sugar Switch on cravings. Ormon's well-written, easy to implement information will take you from feeling sluggish to bursting with energetic vibrancy. Read this book to improve your health and wellbeing. This is a must read book that can change your life exponentially."

> Elaine Lombardi, CHHC, AADP
> Author of Hurricane Lucy: A CAREGIVER'S GUIDE
> Navigating the Storm of Caring for Your Aging Parent

"Cathy Ormon has written a book that is straight from her heart, based on her personal experiences and what she has learned to help her deal with the health challenges she has faced. She has done an incredible amount of research into the various types of foods and how they impact the body, both positively and negatively. After switching to having only positive foods in her meals, she is now passionate about sharing the information that helped her improve her own health so much. The passion shows in her writing."

> Judy Obee

"This information is imperative in todays society where poor diets have contributed to so many health challenges that people are facing. Cathy clearly defines how certain foods affect our physiology and the impact that they have on us on a day to day basis. She lays out the basic steps required to improve our dietary choices and in turn improve our health. This book is a must read for anyone wanting to address their health concerns in a natural way or just looking to improve their overall health."

> Dr. Lynita Haaranen
> Chiropractor

"The Sugar Switch contains excellent information about sugar and its devastating effects on the body. More importantly, Cathy Ormon tells you exactly how to switch off the damage caused by sugar and switch on good health."

> Camille Watson, CHC
> Author of 8 Steps to a Real-Foods Kitchen
> Transform Your Kitchen, Transform Your Health

"The Sugar Switch is an easy to follow guide to healthy lifestyle changes, with a high probability of reaching your goals. Cathy has included a sensible maintenance plan in the Health Coaching Program that matches her book."

> Glen Lewis

"Everyone needs to take a look at their eating habits and what we put into our bodies. There is so much confusing information out there and Cathy helps make sense of it all with The Sugar Switch. As a past client of her program I've learned tips that have changed the way I look at all food. We all deserve the benefit of feeling healthy and understanding how to make positive choices."

> Chrysta Lewis
> Owner, Scarlet Edge Beauty & Esthetics

"Cathy's vast knowledge and her personal journey are inspiring. This book contains imperative information and easy to follow changes you can make in your life to turn off The Sugar Switch for good. I'm starting today!"

> Karen Spencer
> Entrepreneur and Businesswoman, LifeVantage

The Sugar Switch

The Powerful Key to Lose Weight,
Look Good and *Feel Great!*

By Cathy Ormon, CHC. AADP

The Sugar Switch
The Powerful Key to Lose Weight, Look Good and Feel Great!
By Cathy Ormon, CHC, AADP

Copyright © 2015 by Cathy Ormon

The content of this book is for general instruction only. Each person's physical, emotional, and spiritual condition is unique. The instruction in this book is not intended to replace or interrupt the reader's relationship with a physician or other professional. Please consult your doctor for matters pertaining to your specific health and diet.

All rights reserved. No part of this publication may be reproduced, distributed, or transmitted in any form or by any means, including photocopying, recording, or other electronic or mechanical methods, without the prior written permission of the publisher or author, except in the case of brief quotations embodied in critical reviews and certain other noncommercial uses permitted by copyright law.

For permission requests, email the author at:
Cathy@CathyOrmon.com

To contact the author, visit:
www.cathyormon.com

ISBN 978-0-9947441-0-4

Published by:
Cathy Ormon Consulting
Calgary, Alberta, Canada

Printed in the United States of America

Cover Photos (Sugar) by Sid Helischauer, Dynamic Images
Cover Author Photo by Jasmin Poon, Rising Star Productions, Inc.

Book & Cover Design and Graphic Images by Wendy Alessi,
Fig Tree Design Studio

Contents

Praise for The Sugar Switch
Dedication
Acknowledgements
Introduction

Chapter 1: Sugar – Public Enemy #1
    Sugar Consumption is on the Rise
    Refined Sugar and the Confusion of Packaged Food Labels
    The Many Names of Sugar
    About Glucose and Fructose
    Sugar is a Proven Health Hazard

Chapter 2: What is The Sugar Switch?
    The Sugar Switch
    What Flips The Sugar Switch ON?
    What Flips The Sugar Switch OFF?
    What Exactly is Insulin?
    The Sugar Switch ON Scenario: Two Visual Images
    Insulin Resistance
    The Benefits of Controlling The Sugar Switch

Chapter 3: Sugar Switch Triggers
    What are Sugar Switch Triggers?
    Avoid The Sugar Switch Triggers
    The Sugar Switch Triggers List

Chapter 4: The Glycemic Impact of Food
    The Concepts of High Glycemic Food and Low Glycemic Food
        1. Glycemic Index (GI)
        2. Glycemic Load (GL) - Different From Glycemic Index (GI)
    Using the Glycemic Index and Glycemic Load

Contents

Chapter 5: Nutritionally Balanced eating
Is This Just Another Typical Weight-loss Diet?
What is Nutritionally Balanced Eating?
A Simple Daily 4 Step Plan
Meals, Snacks and the Daily 4 Step Plan
The Healthy Food Plate: A Visual of the Daily 4 Step Plan
Reasons For Balanced Meals and Snacks
Remember the Sugar Switch Triggers

Chapter 6: Protein
What is Protein?
Animal Protein versus Vegetable Protein
What is the Best Source of Protein?

Chapter 7: Carbohydrates
What Is a Carbohydrate?
Types of Carbs
Not All Carbohydrates Are Healthy

Chapter 8: Grains
Two Categories of Grains

Chapter 9: Fiber
Startling Fiber Facts
Soluble Fiber
Insoluble Fiber

Chapter 10: Fats – Good versus Harmful
Why Do We Need To Consume Good Fats?
Good Fats
Harmful Fats

Contents

Chapter 11: Water
    Healthy Water is Important
    The Functions of Water
    The Benefits of Drinking Enough Healthy Water
    How Much Water Do We Need?

Chapter 12: Cravings
    What Is a Craving?
    Triggers For Cravings
    Be a Detective! Dig deep...
    Crowding Out: Fill Your World With Healthy Foods and Beverages

Chapter 13: The Physical Connection
    Get Physical!
    Huge Benefits of Physical Activity
    Exercise does not have to be boring
    Exercise Tips and Ideas

Conclusion

List of Related Information:
    Glycemic Load and Glycemic Index
    Insulin Resistance and Metabolic Syndrome
    Memory Loss and Alzheimer's Disease
    Sugar Consumption and Cancer Risk

About the Author

Dedication

This book is dedicated to all of us who are struggling with or have struggled with the effects of sugar and refined foods, with weight issues, with sugar cravings, and with keeping our energy at an optimum level all day long. Know that you are not alone, and there is a natural, totally sustainable way to get your health on track, get rid of excess weight easily, stop the sugar cravings permanently, and have great energy.

Acknowledgements

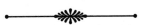

Writing this book has been an incredible experience! I have learned so much and I have been blessed with wonderful people who have helped me in this whole process of becoming a published Author.

I would not have been able to complete this book without my incredible book team. To Elaine Lombardi, Eileen Hartman, Judy Obee, and David Ormon – thank you, thank you, thank you! Your support, good ideas, expert editing skills, and proofreading have been invaluable! Elaine – I appreciate your encouragement and support right from the start. Judy and David - I appreciate your experience, your sharp eyes and your attention to grammar. Judy – I appreciate all your questions, which gave me the push I needed to clarify some of the content, and your patience with the process I was going through. Eileen – I appreciate your experience as an Author, your thoughtful comments throughout the editing process and your attention to small details as well. Special thanks to David for all your loving support of all of my endeavors in health coaching!

I would also like to thank Joshua Rosenthal, Lindsey Smith and the staff at the Institute for Integrative Nutrition (IIN) for their enthusiasm, their support, their guidance and all the wonderful information they give to their students through their courses. It is great to be a part of their vision – creating a world-wide ripple effect of health!

I would like to thank Kristin Dawson for teaching me about the body's insulin production and the concept of low glycemic eating. It was a game changer for me in so many ways, and a springboard to becoming a Health Coach and helping others. Thanks, Kristin!

With much gratitude,

Cathy

Introduction

"The groundwork of all happiness is health."
James Leigh Hunt

Health is our greatest gift. Our health affects absolutely everything we do in life! In order to do the activities we desire and live the life of our dreams – we need to have good, solid health. Without our health, nothing else really matters and we are not happy. I know this to be true from my own experience with a health crash.

Staying healthy is a journey and a learning experience. Most of us are born with good health, and it is definitely something that we take very much for granted. We have always been healthy, so why should that not continue? Our bodies are incredibly miraculous. They are precision machines that have a totally amazing ability to adjust to all sorts of situations, keeping us physically balanced and giving us the energy to be able to do everything we need to do on a daily basis. And this all happens without our being aware of it. We often don't realize that our good health has to be maintained, and that this maintenance needs conscious effort. Staying healthy and learning to maintain our body and our health is a journey all unto itself.

This book is a useful tool that will help you on your health journey. You will learn how sugar affects all of us, through what I call The Sugar Switch. You will also learn how to use the power of good nutrition to control The Sugar Switch, in order to maintain incredible health and energy.

The effects of sugar and The Sugar Switch are not well understood by the majority of people. The Sugar Switch concept involves an important mechanism in our body that is unintentionally abused because of the dietary lifestyle of eating refined foods that we have grown accustomed to consuming. Understanding The Sugar Switch can totally turn your health around, as it did for me.

It is also the powerful key to easy, natural weight loss and increased energy – without weight-loss DIETS.
(The acronym 'DIETS' is explained in Chapter 5)

If you eat the standard North American diet, you are part of a huge population that consumes far too much sugar and highly processed food. Over many decades, we have steadily veered away from the wholesome, nutrient rich food of our forefathers.

In our modern, western society, we are surrounded by clever marketing 24 hours per day, 7 days per week. There seems to be no escape – even the wide-open spaces of the Alberta foothills have large billboards along the Trans-Canada Highway. The marketers are very effective. Highly processed food is the subject of much of the advertising - whether on television, on billboards, in newspapers, online ads, or flyers that come to the door.
The marketing is often misleading because it uses catchy words that are ambiguous and it leads us to believe that all of these highly processed foods are somehow good for us. The advertising contains catch phrases that are so convincing that we inevitably become interested in the products.

The fact is that most of this fast, convenient, processed food is totally void of beneficial nutrients and is harmful to our health. Unbeknownst to most people - these foods are actually toxic to our body.

Throughout the pages of this book you will learn which foods to completely avoid, which foods to consume in moderation, which foods to consume daily, and why. The Sugar Switch is something that everyone has complete control over - simply by choosing the foods that are consumed.

This book is a guide to getting back to the basics of eating whole foods, fresh vegetables and fruits. It is an important educational piece of the weight loss puzzle that is missing. This book is not another typical weight loss diet. Rather, this book is about choosing a healthy, nutritional lifestyle. It is based on making small, sustainable changes in daily food choices.

It is all about gaining the knowledge to move steadfastly forward, towards a healthy, whole foods lifestyle.

This book lays out a basic, no nonsense blueprint for you to follow, which guides you to steadily lose weight without another typical weight loss diet. Using this blueprint you will be able to lose weight easily, and kick the carb or sugar cravings. You will notice increased energy, and you will be substantially reducing your risk for common, chronic diseases such as diabetes, obesity, high blood pressure, high cholesterol, fatty liver, heart issues, joint pain, inflammation and much more.

I am passionate about helping people understand how to achieve great health and energy – by consciously making healthy choices. My purpose in writing this book is to help people recover from the negative effects of sugar and refined foods, and to tell people that getting rid of excess weight, stopping the sugar and carb cravings and gaining energy can be a simple, natural process. This book incorporates my own personal experience from my health journey, knowledge from my Health Coach education as well as research I have done, and the experience of coaching numerous clients to successfully learn about and control their Sugar Switch.

I sincerely wish you the best in your health journey. May this book be a guiding light and a blessing on your way!

Chapter 1: Sugar - Public Enemy #1

Sugar Consumption is on the Rise

Sweets and sweet flavors are a part of our North American culture, but we seem to be going completely overboard with the amount of sugar we are consuming. And that amount seems to be increasing every year. Excess sugar consumption, particularly certain harmful sugars and chemical sweeteners are undermining our health in a big way. Sugar is definitely Public Enemy #1.

Sugar has become an addiction for us, due to our over consumption of refined foods. Consuming too much junk food and highly processed carbohydrates causes relentless cravings and perpetuates the addiction. This forces us into a vicious circle that is never ending. Even more sugar is consumed because it is hidden in products that are touted as being healthy. The overabundance of sugar we are consuming has become a health hazard.

Sweets have a chemical effect on our brain causing the brain to release serotonin and dopamine, our body's feel good chemicals. Given that fact, it makes sense that comfort food – foods that people have connected with a feeling of being comforted or feeling loved or stress relief – are very often refined, sweet foods, high in sugar content like donuts, cake, cookies, chocolate bars, etc. We rarely hear of vegetables such as broccoli being consumed as a comfort food, even though there is some natural sugar in vegetables.

Refined Sugar and the Confusion of Packaged Food Labels

Refined sugar is in almost everything. Sugar is used by food manufacturers to make processed foods taste good, so that people will develop a liking for them and continue to buy them.

Because our tastes have been attuned to the super sweetness from sugars in all the refined foods we are consuming, we seem to have forgotten just how naturally sweet fresh fruits and vegetables really are.

When we read the Food Nutrition Facts on a packaged food product, we are not sure if the grams of sugar listed comes from a healthy natural source, such as from a piece of fruit, or if it comes from added refined sugar that is totally unnecessary.

And the terms used on packaged goods (which are generally regulated by government agencies) can also be misleading. Take, for example the terms "sugar free" or "no sugar": this doesn't mean that there is zero sugar; it means that food products can contain up to 0.5 grams of sugar AND contain less than 5 calories per specified serving size. The keywords 'free', 'zero' or 'without' mean the food contains a small amount of a nutrient, such as sugar, which is deemed not to have any effect on the body.

The Many Names of Sugar

Yes, sugar seems to be hiding in everything that is processed. We eat a significant amount of refined sugar every day, without even realizing it. Many people think of candy, cakes, donuts and baked goods as the main source of refined sugar. But the truth is that sugar is hidden in almost all processed foods – foods that seem to be healthy and not sweet including sauces, dressings, ketchup, marinades, crackers, cereals, breads, cheese spreads and even baby formula.

Natural sweeteners:

Important note: Consuming ANY type of added sugar or sweetener (even natural sweeteners) in excess amounts is not healthy.

There are many different types of natural sweeteners, which are not refined derivatives of sugar itself. Make no mistake – they are sweeteners, but some of them have nutritional value, which gives them some health benefit, and some do not. Some of these natural sweeteners are not as harmful to the body, and some of them are harmful:

Maple syrup - from maple trees; has nutritional value; much less harmful than refined sugar.

Agave syrup - from a cactus plant; has no nutritional value; can be very harmful.

Stevia - a herbal plant; has no nutritional value; is not harmful.

Xylitol - from trees or corn husks; has no nutritional value; much less harmful than refined sugar.

Date sugar - from dates; has nutritional value; is not harmful

Coconut sugar - from the coconut palm; has some nutritional value; much less harmful than refined sugar.

Honey - from bee nectar; has nutritional value; much less harmful than refined sugar.

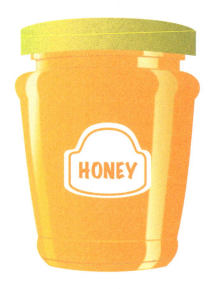

Refined sugar

Refined sugar itself has so many forms and names that we, the consumer, find it totally confusing. When reading the ingredients list of a product, we find it difficult to figure out which of those ingredients actually mean refined sugar. And some of the names for refined sugar are misleading because they sound healthier than they really are, like 'concentrated fruit juice'.

Here are some of the names used for refined sugar: (not a complete list)

- Barley Malt
- Beet sugar
- Black strap molasses
- Brown rice syrup
- Brown sugar
- Buttered sugar
- Cane juice
- Cane sugar
- Caramel
- Carob syrup
- Castor sugar
- Concentrated fruit juice
- Confectioner's sugar
- Corn sweetener
- Corn syrup
- Crystalline fructose
- Demerara sugar
- Diastatic malt
- Diatase
- Dextran
- Ethyl maltol
- Evaporated cane juice
- Fructose
- Fruit juice concentrates
- Galactose
- Glucose
- Golden sugar
- Golden syrup
- High fructose corn syrup (HFCS)
- Invert sugar
- Lactose
- Malt syrup
- Maltodextrin
- Maltose
- Molasses syrup
- Muscovado sugar
- Organic raw sugar
- Oat syrup
- Panela
- Panocha
- Rice bran syrup
- Rice syrup
- Sorghum
- Sorghum syrup
- Sugar
- Syrup
- Tapioca syrup
- Turbinado sugar
- Yellow sugar

About Glucose and Fructose

Sugar or sucrose consists of two simple sugars: glucose and fructose. They are both sugars, but they are different, particularly in terms of how the body metabolizes them.

Glucose is vital to life and is found in all cells. Our body produces it. It is also found in starches such as potatoes. Glucose can be used by every cell in our body. It is the energy or fuel that we were designed to use.

Fructose is not produced by the body. It is found in fruits and vegetables, and in added processed or refined sugars.

Important note: The fructose in fruits and vegetables is not harmful because the fruit and vegetables contain other nutritional elements such as fiber, vitamins and minerals. The fructose that we derive from these whole foods is minimal in our standard North American diet compared to the fructose we consume from refined added sugars. Fructose and HFCS (high fructose corn syrup) are the two main forms of refined sugar used by most food manufacturers.

Fructose in the form of processed sugar is very harmful. Why? The only organ in our body that can metabolize fructose in significant amounts is the liver. If the liver becomes overloaded with fructose, it turns the fructose into fat. This fat ends up as elevated blood triglycerides, bad cholesterol, fat around the organs (and other parts of the body), fatty liver, and the excess fat can cause heart disease.

Sugar Is a Proven Health Hazard

Sugar damages our body in so many ways! Most of us are not even aware of the negative effects of high sugar consumption. Sugar has been linked to countless chronic illnesses, including cancer.

Here are 10 reasons why sugar is harmful to your health. Some of these reasons are fairly obvious, and some may surprise you:

1. Blood sugar rollercoaster: Sugar causes the elevation of blood sugar, excess insulin production, and then a sudden drop in blood sugar. This is known as the blood sugar rollercoaster. We will be covering this subject at length later in this book as we learn more about The Sugar Switch.

2. Insulin resistance: Consuming high amounts of refined sugar causes insulin resistance, meaning that the body no longer responds properly to the insulin that it produces, with the end result being diabetes and obesity. This can contribute to many chronic diseases. There is a link between insulin resistance and The Sugar Switch.

3. An empty food: Refined sugar does not contain any nutrients, enzymes, protein, fiber or healthy fats. It is void of all nutrients – an empty food! There is nothing in refined sugar to slow down its absorption into the blood as blood sugar, and there is nothing to give us the feeling that we are full or that we need to stop eating the empty foods. In nutrient dense foods, the fiber and protein give us the feeling of fullness, so we can regulate our food intake. This means that many people tend to overeat on sugary items and don't realize it.

4. Leading cause of heart disease: Sugar has recently been shown to be a leading cause of heart disease. Fructose, a major component of many highly refined foods, is the culprit because it raises the major risk factors for heart disease: increased blood glucose levels, insulin levels, LDL (bad) cholesterol, oxidized LDL cholesterol (very bad), triglycerides and increased abdominal obesity.

5. It is addictive: It can cause massive amounts of dopamine to be released in the brain, which can lead to addiction.

6. Accelerates aging: After sugar enters the blood stream it can attach to proteins in a process known as glycation. These newly formed cells contribute to loss of elasticity in tissues and organs. This can lead to premature aging and can cause the skin to become saggy or wrinkly.

7. Damages cognitive health: According to Dr. Joseph Mercola, recent studies are showing that higher blood sugar levels have a negative impact on the brain's cognitive ability. The theory is that high blood sugar causes high insulin levels, which can disrupt signals to the brain and damage cognitive ability.

8. Increases stress: Excess sugar consumption causes the body to release the fight or flight hormones adrenalin, noradrenaline and cortisol. While these hormones give the body a burst of energy, they can also cause a feeling of anxiousness.

9. Affects the immune system: Sugar can suppress the body's immune system by affecting the balance of yeast and bacteria in the body. Since bacteria and yeast feed off of sugar, excess sugar can cause the bacteria and yeast to overgrow and become unbalanced. Infections and illness are more likely when the bacteria and yeast are out of balance.

10. Linked to cancer: There is mounting evidence that high consumption of sugar and sugary refined foods may be linked to a risk of various types of cancer, including breast, colon and pancreatic cancer. (See the List of Related Information at the back of the book.)

Chapter 2: What is The Sugar Switch?

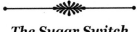

The Sugar Switch

The Sugar Switch is what I decided to name the body's excess production of insulin. I chose this name because it is visual, calling to mind a switch on a wall – like a light switch. We all know how to flip a switch to turn a light on or off. We can do a very similar flip of a switch inside our body to turn our body's excess production of insulin ON or OFF, even though we cannot see the switch or touch it.

For the purposes of this book – the terms blood sugar and blood glucose have the same meaning: sugar in the blood.

When your Sugar Switch is flipped ON – your body is forced to produce excess insulin to deal with excess sugar in your blood. This is not a healthy situation. When your Sugar Switch is flipped OFF – your body's insulin production is not excessive and not forced. Your body has a normal insulin response that is healthy. In fact, when your Sugar Switch is OFF your body will automatically produce glucagon – a fat burning hormone.

What Flips The Sugar Switch ON?

In general, certain types of foods and beverages will flip The Sugar Switch ON: highly refined foods, junk food, sugary foods and beverages, alcohol, foods that fill our tummies but have no nutritional value for us.

Why do these foods flip The Sugar Switch ON? These foods are highly processed and/or contain high amounts of sugar. They digest very quickly, turning to blood sugar very quickly and enter the blood stream fast, in a large quantity. So the blood stream is flooded with blood sugar, which prompts the body to flip The Sugar Switch ON and produce excess insulin in order to deal with the blood sugar overload.

What Flips The Sugar Switch OFF?

The Sugar Switch is flipped OFF by having a healthy, balanced, whole foods lifestyle – which means eating foods that contain the nutrition your body needs. For the most part, these foods are either minimally processed or totally unprocessed.

Why do these foods flip The Sugar Switch OFF? Healthy, nutritionally dense whole foods contain nutrients that the body needs, such as fiber, that slow down the digestion of food. When the food digests slowly, it turns into blood sugar more slowly, and enters the blood stream at a slower, more even rate. The blood stream does not become flooded with blood sugar, so the body does not need to produce excess insulin. The Sugar Switch is, in effect, switched OFF.

What Exactly is Insulin?

Insulin is a fat storing hormone with an extremely important job to do in keeping us healthy. Your body must maintain a balanced level of sugar in the blood at all times, and insulin is the hormone that keeps that balance.

Here's a short and broad explanation of how it works: when you eat, your food is digested and during the digestive process it turns to sugar and enters your bloodstream. This is called blood sugar or blood glucose. Your body responds by producing insulin. Insulin is absolutely necessary to take the blood sugar out of the blood and transport it to the cells for energy. Insulin effectively unlocks the cells, so the blood sugar / glucose can enter. The glucose is then stored in the cells and used for energy later, when needed.

The Sugar Switch ON Scenario –Two Visual Images

There are two visual images that can be used to explain the negative cycle that happens when The Sugar Switch is ON: The Blood Sugar Rollercoaster, and The Vicious Circle.

Visual Image 1: The Blood Sugar Rollercoaster

Consuming highly processed foods, sugary foods, alcohol and junk foods will cause a chain reaction that is like a sharp rollercoaster. Here is a graph that illustrates how your blood sugar level varies over time, depending on what you have eaten.

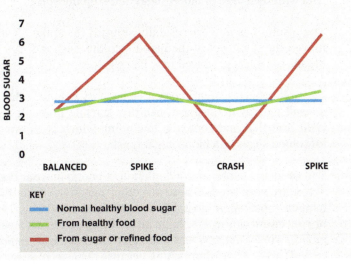

- At the starting point, the blood sugar rollercoaster is in the normal, healthy, middle zone (the blue line in the chart above), not too high and not too low - right where it should be. Athletes sometimes call this the *performance zone* because the body's energy is even and continuous.

- Highly refined foods, sugar or junk food are consumed. They digest very quickly, turning into blood sugar rapidly.

- You experience a surge of energy in your body from the rising blood sugar (the red line in the chart). This is the rollercoaster on a fast, steep climb to a peak, known as a blood sugar spike.

- The excess blood sugar and fast, steep spike has flipped The Sugar Switch ON.

- Your body responds quickly by producing excess insulin to deal with the surge of blood sugar and stop the spike.

- The insulin has now successfully stopped the spike. It has moved the sugar out of the blood – to the cells, muscles or organs (or it has produced new fat cells to store it in).

- The rollercoaster then starts a steep, fast decline. But it doesn't stop at the normal, healthy, starting point. It zips right past that and goes to a low point, which is known as low blood sugar or a blood sugar crash.

- You suddenly experience a depletion of energy in your body – you are very tired. There are other negative effects that happen most often: irritability, brain fog, headache, lack of concentration, jitters, light headedness or feeling weak, mood swings, hunger, and you start craving sugar or processed carbs. This is happening because the level of sugar in the blood is very low.

- You automatically respond by eating something so that you can quickly feel better. What you automatically reach for is something sweet, something highly processed so that you have energy again – and fast!

- The rollercoaster starts all over again – quickly climbing to a spike and turning ON The Sugar Switch, forcing more insulin to be produced, getting blood sugar out of the blood, then a blood sugar crash, then the craving. It repeats over and over again.

- This rollercoaster effect happens repeatedly every day, creating many health issues over time.

Visual Image 2: The Vicious Circle

The fast rise and fall of blood sugar can also be seen as a vicious circle that goes round and round and round.

This is a different way of illustrating the same scenario:
- eating highly refined foods forces the body to produce excess insulin (a fat storing hormone).
- The Sugar Switch is now ON and the blood sugar spikes.
- blood sugar is transferred to cells or stored as fat.
- blood sugar has now been removed from the blood causing a low blood sugar crash.
- this results in negative effects in the body (low energy, mood swings, hunger, irritability, etc.)
- then the cravings start – a physical urge to eat more sugar, a need for a quick fix for low blood sugar; the vicious circle starts all over again with highly refined foods. On and on it goes!

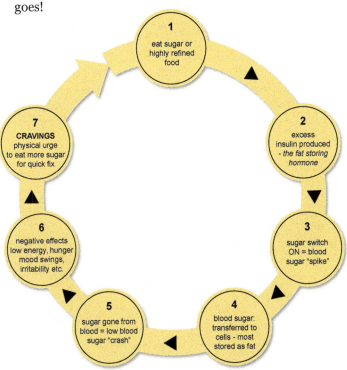

Insulin Resistance

When The Sugar Switch is always ON and the body is forced to continually produce excess insulin because of poor dietary choices (highly processed foods, sugar and junk foods), the cells eventually stop reacting to the insulin. At that point, the insulin's ability to unlock the cells becomes impaired, so your cells stop accepting the blood sugar as energy. In response, your body must produce more and more insulin to deal with the blood sugar and maintain a balance.

Remember that the blood sugar must be kept balanced in order for your body to be healthy. When the cells stop reacting to the insulin and do not open to accept blood sugar, the body has a challenge and has to find a way to get the sugar out of the blood. So, it either has to store the sugar in the muscles or an organ, primarily the liver, or it has to make more cells to store the sugar in. The new cells it makes are fat cells. Thus, insulin is a fat storing hormone.

This is a very unhealthy situation known as insulin resistance, with many negative health effects. Insulin resistance results in high triglyceride levels, high blood pressure, pre-diabetes and diabetes, and obesity. Insulin resistance can also lead to heart disease.

Insulin resistance is very serious because it can cause so many other chronic health issues. The good news is that insulin resistance is usually completely reversible.

The Benefits of Controlling The Sugar Switch

1. You will tame the carb/sugar cravings **permanently** when you learn how to control your Sugar Switch by turning it OFF. Junk food and sweets will no longer be controlling you! In fact, you will most likely find that sugary and sweet foods are *too* sweet and they no longer appeal to you.

2. Your body's blood sugar level will remain balanced, in the middle zone (also known by athletes as the *performance zone*) where the body burns fat (your blood sugar is not spiking and not crashing).

3. You will be keeping your body's metabolism burning evenly throughout the day, (in the *performance zone*), which gives you energy to do everything you want to do – all day long.

4. Your body will not gain weight because it will not be producing excess insulin, which is the fat storing hormone. You will be able to enjoy guilt-free eating and weight-loss diets will be a thing of the past.

5. If you are overweight, your body will be able to release the weight it needs to lose without any effort. There is no need to count calories or weigh your food. You will look good and feel great!

6. You will no longer have the negative effects associated with sugar cravings and low blood sugar: mood swings, brain fog, irritability, jitters, headaches, lack of concentration, light headedness or feeling weak, and mid-afternoon energy slumps.

7. Risk factors for metabolic syndrome and common chronic health issues will naturally decrease. This includes risk factors for: obesity, diabetes, high blood pressure, high triglyceride levels, high LDL (bad) cholesterol levels, inflammation, fatty liver, and more.

8. Your body will be getting good, healthy nutrition when you control your Sugar Switch through eating the right kind of carbohydrates, in the form of whole foods that are full of beneficial nutrients (instead of choosing carbs from refined junk foods that are nutritionally empty).

Chapter 3: Sugar Switch Triggers

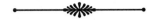

What Are Sugar Switch Triggers?

Sugar Switch triggers are foods that cause the rollercoaster effect of blood sugar spikes and crashes, and they are harmful to your health. They are foods that are quickly digested, turning into blood sugar very fast, which causes the blood sugar to spike, and forces the body to produce excess insulin to deal with the excess blood sugar.

Sugar Switch triggers can be put into five basic categories:

1. Sugar. Sugar has many forms and names, and it is hidden in many refined foods that otherwise might seem like healthy choices (see Chapter 1). The obvious examples of sugar are candy bars, cookies, baked goods. Some less obvious examples where sugar is hidden are sauces, condiments, and beverages.

2. Empty foods. Most Sugar Switch triggers are foods that have little or no fiber, and most often have very few nutrients (or none at all), which makes them empty foods. Example: white breads, bagels and wheat-based pasta.

3. Foods naturally high in sugar. There are some Sugar Switch triggers that contain some nutrients but also contain a large amount of natural sugar. These foods can trigger the blood sugar to spike and crash. Dried fruit is an example of this, even if the fruit is not soaked in a sugar solution before being dried.

4. Additives. Some foods start out as healthy foods, but they become Sugar Switch triggers because of the processing or refining they have been put through. Additives have been put into them, which turns them into Sugar Switch triggers.

Ham is a good example because it has a high amount of sugar and salt added during the curing process. Ham is also high in nitrates, which are unhealthy.

5. Alcohol. Alcoholic beverages will turn to sugar and enter the bloodstream very quickly when they are consumed without healthy, balanced food.

Some Sugar Switch triggers can be modified to slow down the rate of digestion and absorption into the blood stream. Some Sugar Switch triggers are very harmful and really cannot be modified - they will have to be permanently deleted from daily dietary intake. In some cases, protein and fiber will slow down the process. Consuming a small amount of a Sugar Switch trigger (versus consuming a large quantity) can also be a factor in slowing down the process.

Avoid The Sugar Switch Triggers

For 45 to 60 days (perhaps up to 90 days, depending upon the individual person) there are some Sugar Switch trigger foods that you MUST stop eating in order to control The Sugar Switch and transition from your current refined foods lifestyle to a healthier whole foods lifestyle. After this period of time – most of these foods can be added back in, *with modifications.* A few of the foods, the harmful foods, will need to be deleted from your whole foods lifestyle *permanently.*

An overview: 3 categories within The Sugar Switch triggers list:

- ***Permanently deleted foods:*** Some foods are unhealthy and will cause damage to your health. These foods need to be deleted permanently.

- ***Temporarily deleted foods:*** Some foods need to be deleted temporarily during the transition from your current eating lifestyle to a new healthier whole foods lifestyle. These foods can be added back in with important and permanent modifications when a whole foods, low glycemic lifestyle has been successfully incorporated.

- ***Foods to keep, with modifications:*** Some foods are okay to eat right from the beginning, but need to have modifications.

Bio-individuality is important!

- The exact amount of time these foods will be limited depends upon the individual person. For people who have the goal of getting rid of a large amount of weight - it is best to use the 60 day guideline. For people with a minimal amount of weight to get rid of - the 45 day guideline might be the best.

- Also consider other modifications based on any allergies or sensitivities you might have, such as gluten, nuts, dairy or soy. You are the person who knows your body best.

The Sugar Switch Triggers List

Permanently delete these foods and beverages:

SUGARS:
   Permanently replace sugar with small quantities of stevia, xylitol, berries or fruit to sweeten.

COMMERCIAL JUICES and SWEETENED BEVERAGES and ALL SOFT DRINKS:
   All commercial juices, iced teas and sweetened beverages. This includes ALL soft drinks (even the diet, sugar free, or zero calorie ones). Exception: tomato juice is okay in limited quantities (due to it's high salt content).

DEEP FRIED FOODS:
   ALL deep fried foods!

CERTAIN DAIRY and ALL RICE MILKS/BEVERAGES:
   ALL 0% fat dairy products, skim milk and rice milk.

Here are the reasons:
- 0% dairy products have the fat taken out and it is replaced by other unhealthy ingredients such as sugar.

- Our body needs some fat, which could come from healthier 2% dairy products instead.

- Rice milk is made from highly processed rice and will spike blood sugar very quickly.

REFINED JUNK FOODS, SNACKS and FAST FOODS:
Foods that are totally refined and contain no nutrients (or extremely small amount of nutrients) fill up our tummy but leave us nutritionally starving. This includes pretzels, fries, chips and related products, commercial baked goods, candies, commercial pizza, fast foods found in the freezer section of any food store - the list goes on and on. Rule of thumb: if it is a refined fast food, it has probably been processed to the point of no nutrition in order to make it into a fast food.

Temporarily Deleted Foods:

Temporarily delete these items from your daily food choices (45 to 60 days). They can be added back in when a whole foods, low glycemic lifestyle has been successfully incorporated. The *permanent modifications* are in parentheses.

POTATOES:
Can be added back in later, with important and *permanent modifications* (baby potatoes instead of large baking potatoes and NO breaded or deep fried potatoes).

DRIED FRUITS:
Can be added back in later, with important and *permanent modifications* (need to consume enough fiber and protein with the dried fruit).

MEAT:
Ham – can be added back in later (consume in small quantities only).

CORN:
   Can be added back in later, with important and *permanent modifications*. (consume in small quantities only)

GRAINS (wheat, rice and other grains):
   Can be added back in later, with important and *permanent modifications*. (MUST be whole grains – not refined grains. NO white flour products. NO white rice. Must be consumed in limited quantities.)

BEER, WINE and ALCOHOLIC BEVERAGES:
   Can be added back in later, with important and *permanent modifications*. (Consume in small quantities only; NOT to be consumed by itself without food; consume with balanced and nutritious food only – NOT junk food.)
   NOTE: Soft drinks should not be consumed at all – they are extremely hazardous to your health!

Foods to keep, but *MUST have modifications***:**

HOMEMADE JUICES:
   MUST have vegetables combined with fruit (NOT just fruit).

FRIED FOODS:
   Consume very limited quantities of fried foods, using only coconut oil (for high heat) or olive oil (for moderate heat). NO deep fried foods.

DAIRY:
   2% milk, 2% plain Greek yogurt (NOT flavored), limited amounts of high fat cheese, although cheese that has lower Milk Fat (MF) is okay. Unsweetened soy or almond milk is okay. NO rice milk of any kind.

MEAT:
   All lean meats (except ham), not meats with high fat content. Other recommended modification: organic, hormone free, or free range.

Chapter 4: The Glycemic Impact of Food

The Concepts of High Glycemic Food and Low Glycemic Food

There are two tools to indicate whether a food is high glycemic or low glycemic: Glycemic Index, known as GI, and Glycemic Load, known as GL.

High glycemic food is a phrase that refers to any food that has a high glycemic index (GI) number or glycemic load (GL) number. High glycemic food will spike the blood sugar very quickly, causing the whole process of too much insulin, excess fat being stored, and many negative effects on the body (the rollercoaster or vicious circle effects as illustrated in Chapter 2.).

Low glycemic food refers to any food that has a low GI or GL number. Low glycemic food will digest more slowly and not spike your blood sugar quickly, unless you eat an unhealthy, large quantity of it at one time. Choosing to consume low glycemic foods will keep your blood sugar in the healthy middle zone and it will not cause all the negative effects of too much insulin production.

Glycemic impact is the overall effect or impact that a food or combination of foods has on blood sugar. As you will see below in both glycemic index and glycemic load, there are certain factors that influence the glycemic impact of carbohydrates.

1. Glycemic Index (GI)

The Glycemic index, often referred to as GI, was a new concept introduced in the early 1980's by Dr. David Jenkins, University of Toronto. It is a numerical system designed to rate how fast carbohydrate foods are broken down into glucose and enter the blood stream as they are digested by the body.

Dr. Jenkins assigned a GI number of 100 to glucose and set that as the standard. All other carbs are measured, rated and compared to that standard.

The GI number of a carb gives us an idea of **how fast** that particular carb will **TURN ON our Sugar Switch** by spiking or raising our blood sugar. This is valuable information for all of us, but especially for diabetics.

GI numbers fall into 3 categories:
    1. **Low GI:** under 55 (not as fast to turn Sugar Switch ON)
    2. **Medium GI:** 55 – 70 (turns ON Sugar Switch fast)
    3. **High GI:** over 70 (turns ON Sugar Switch extremely fast)

Five factors that influence a carbohydrate's GI number and the glycemic impact:

1. How ripe a food is (example: very brown bananas have a higher glycemic impact than not-so-ripe yellow bananas)

2. How processed the carbohydrate is (example: bleached white flour has a very high glycemic impact).

3. Cooking: how the food was cooked and/or the length of time the food has been cooked (foods that have been cooked for a long period of time are often higher glycemic).

4. How much fiber a carbohydrate contains (high fiber foods have a lower glycemic impact).

5. The amount of sugar the carbohydrate contains (carbohydrates with a higher sugar content have a higher glycemic impact).

But wait! THERE'S MORE: the GI number is not enough information – it does NOT take into consideration the quantity of the carbohydrate, so it is not a complete picture for us. The Glycemic Load is a more accurate indicator.

2. Glycemic Load (GL) - Different from Glycemic Index (GI)

The Glycemic Load is often referred to as GL. It is different from the GI number. The GL number is a **more important indicator** than the GI number because it gives a more accurate assessment of how fast a carb will TURN ON The Sugar Switch.

The GL takes into consideration both the *quantity and the quality of the carbohydrate* because both are factors that affect how fast a carbohydrate turns to glucose in our bodies. The GI number by itself only looks at half of the equation, so it can be deceiving (see the example below).

GL numbers fall into three categories:
   1. Low GL: 0 – 10 (very, very slow to turn ON The Sugar Switch)
   2. Medium GL: 10 – 20 (slow to turn ON The Sugar Switch)
   3. High GL: over 20 (will easily turn ON The Sugar Switch)

Figuring out the GL number – a formula to use:

There is a formula to determine the glycemic load of a food. Knowing this formula is helpful because most information using the low glycemic concept only states the glycemic index number. Here is the formula to use:

- the food's glycemic index number (GI) multiplied by the number of grams of carbohydrates per serving, divided by 100

OR

   (GI number X carbohydrate grams/serving) divided by 100 = Glycemic Load

Here is a very good example that illustrates how deceiving it can be when only the GI number is considered. The example is taken from the book Healthy for Life by Dr. Ray Strand.

Looking at *only the glycemic index (GI) number:*

- One cup of **cooked pasta** has a **GI of 41** (and contains 52 g of carbohydrates).

- An average serving of **carrots** (about ½ cup) has a **GI of 49** (and contains 5 g of carbohydrates).

- GI of 41 for the pasta versus GI of 49 for the carrots. So – it looks like the pasta is a better choice because it has a lower GI number, right? WRONG!

Now let's *look at the glycemic load (GL) of each of the same foods:*

- One cup of **cooked pasta** has a **GL of 21.3**, which is HIGH. (41 GI X 52 grams of carbs = 2132, divided by 100 = 21.3 GL).

- An average serving of **carrots** (about ½ cup) has a **GL of 2.45,** which is LOW (49 GI X 5 grams of carbs = 245 divided by 100 = 2.45 GL)

- **Therefore the carrots have a lower glycemic load**

Four factors that can lower the GL of a carbohydrate and the glycemic impact:

1. consuming enough protein with the food
2. consuming enough fiber with the food
3. consuming the food along with some acidic foods (such as lemon juice, pickles, etc.)
4. reducing the food's portion size / eating less of the food

Using the Glycemic Index and Glycemic Load

The goal of a healthy whole foods lifestyle is to learn about and consume whole foods that nourish the body, give you energy, stop cravings, normalize body weight, and support your mental and physical health – now and in the future (permanently), so you can sustain good health in the long term.

Understanding the whole glycemic index and glycemic load concept can help you do this. Foods and beverages that are high glycemic are very unhealthy and can cause major health issues. Foods and beverages that are low glycemic keep your metabolism and blood sugar operating at peak performance, and have a chain reaction of positive health effects.

How can you use GI and GL to permanently maintain a healthier lifestyle, gain energy and maintain your ideal body weight?

How to use GI and GL as guiding tools: 7 Steps

1. Understand the concept of high and low glycemic foods, and glycemic impact. Know the difference between GI and GL. Remember that glycemic load is the best indicator because it accounts for quantity of the carbohydrate in the food as well as quality.

2. You will need to learn how to use the formula to convert the GI number of a carbohydrate food into the GL number for that food. Often the GI number is available for a carbohydrate, but the GL number might not be available. Here is the conversion formula again:
   - Take the carbohydrate's GI number, multiply by the number of grams of carbohydrates per serving, then divide by 100. (see examples earlier in this chapter)

3. Know the low, medium and high number ranges for glycemic load:
    - Low GL is 0 to 10 (medium low would be between 5 and 10)
    - Medium GL is 11 to 20 (medium high would be between 15 and 20)
    - High GL is over 20

4. Know specifically which foods are high glycemic (generally: highly processed, deep fried, sugary, junk foods with no nutrition) and which foods are low glycemic (generally: whole foods – fresh fruits, vegetables, whole unprocessed grains that contain nutrition).
    - There is a list of List of Related Information at the end of this book.
    - Foods and beverages that have a low GL are the foods that will not spike blood sugar, unless a person consumes a huge amount of them at one time.
    - So, your best plan would be to consume whole foods and healthy beverages that are low glycemic.

5. Know that proteins generally do not have a GI or GL number, unless they also contain carbohydrates.
    - Meat, fish and poultry do not have a GI or GL number.
    - Nuts are both a protein and a carbohydrate, so they have a GI and GL number.
    - Consuming enough protein with a carbohydrate is one of the ways to lower the glycemic impact of a food.

6. When cooking, look for and use recipes that you determine are low glycemic, or adjust an existing recipe to be low glycemic.
    - Example of adjusting a recipe: if you are making pancakes or biscuits – take out the high glycemic white processed wheat flour and add in a mixture of healthier flours such as buckwheat flour, quinoa flour, chickpea flour, amaranth flour or almond flour. These healthier flours contain protein and fiber, which will lower the glycemic impact of the pancakes or biscuits.

7. Always make healthy, low glycemic dietary choices, whether you are cooking your own food or you are dining out.
   - Remember that certain sugar trigger foods need to be permanently deleted from your whole foods lifestyle. This includes all refined sugars, commercial juices and sweetened beverages, refined junk foods and snacks, deep fried foods, certain dairy products and rice milk.

Chapter 5: Nutritionally Balanced Eating

Is This Just Another Typical Weight-loss Diet?

Great question! The answer is - no, this is not another typical weight-loss diet!

An extremely important note: there is a very big difference between a typical weight-loss DIET and a healthy whole foods lifestyle that is nutritionally balanced. I believe that typical weight-loss diets are 'DIETS' (singular: DIET), which stands for **D**o **I**t **E**xactly **T**his way with **S**hort-term results.

For the purposes of this book, *healthy whole foods lifestyle* means consuming whole foods with beneficial nutrients that help us maintain good health and energy.

DIETS (typical weight-loss diets):

- are not designed as a healthy, permanent lifestyle.
- are not sustainable: they are designed to work for only a short time.
- tell people exactly what to eat for a temporary period of time.
- most often do not have a healthy balance of nutritional elements, which can have side effects such as headaches, cravings, continuous hunger, jitters, brain fog, irritability and energy crashes from low blood sugar.
- do not educate people on the principles of healthy nutrition.
- do not educate people about how to successfully maintain healthy nutrition and eat for long-term success.
- are often built on guilt, not positive learning and positive changes.
- after a DIET, people very often regain the weight they lost and more! This is because there has been no education about nutrition, how to make small, sustainable, healthy changes, and how to live with a healthy, nutritious whole foods lifestyle.

What is a healthy whole foods lifestyle?

I define a healthy whole foods lifestyle as combining positive knowledge about nutrition, how food affects the body, and how food affects you as a unique individual. With this knowledge, you will have the power to make healthier choices and feel great!

A healthy whole foods lifestyle:

Is all about
- positive learning and building new, healthy habits – with no guilt!
- making a sustainable transition from a harmful, refined foods lifestyle, to a healthy, whole foods lifestyle.
- freedom to make good food choices, which have great health benefits.

Is based on
- the principles of healthy, whole foods nutrition.
- knowledge of harmful foods to avoid, and what makes these foods so harmful.
- knowledge of foods that are healthy and why they should be part of daily nutrition.

Is sustainable because
- it is anchored to a foundation of good nutritional principles that you will be able to use on a daily basis.
- whole foods are incorporated in manageable steps, over a period of time.

Has 3 major long term benefits:
- increases energy and vitality.
- reduces or eliminates the risk of many common chronic illnesses including overweight and obesity.
- reduces or eliminates cravings - permanently.

Is long term, with permanent results and permanent weight loss.

In order to build new healthy habits, learn and move toward a healthier whole foods lifestyle, a person has to STOP the unhealthy dietary habits they currently have. Change cannot take place without this process: the unhealthy dietary habits must be stopped and new, healthy food habits must be learned and incorporated. It might seem in the beginning that what is suggested here is like a DIET. But rest assured – it is NOT a DIET! It is the exercise of forming a new, healthy, whole foods lifestyle.

It can take up to 6 weeks to learn and make a transition towards a new, healthy, whole foods lifestyle. Depending upon the individual person and the amount of weight that will be coming off, it could more time - possibly up to 12 weeks or slightly longer. The learning itself takes time, and building new healthy habits takes time. Statistics show that it takes about 28 days to build a new habit.

Your keys to success are:
- willingness to learn good nutritional principles
- a desire to improve your health by making good, healthy food choices
- a commitment to make this a permanent lifestyle change.

What is nutritionally balanced eating?

Your body needs certain nutritional elements every day in order to function properly, beginning at the cellular level. Nutrition affects every aspect of your life including your energy, your thinking, your body weight, your movement and the functions of all your major organs.

Nutritionally balanced eating is making sure that every meal and every snack contain nutritional elements that support your health and keep your blood sugar in the middle zone (not spiking and not crashing).

A Simple Daily 4 Step Plan

There is a simple Daily 4 Step Plan. It consists of 4 nutritional elements in every meal and every snack, every day. Why the 4 elements?
- To keep your metabolism burning
- To provide you with constant energy
- To keep you from being too hungry
- To prevent having low blood sugar between meals

There will be more specific information about the 4 elements in subsequent chapters.

The 4 Steps are:

1. Protein: consume 15-20 grams per meal; and 8-10 grams per snack. Choose a healthy protein source.

2. Fiber: consume 8-10 grams per meal and 4-6 grams per snack. Obtain fiber from good carbohydrates that are mainly found in 3 food categories:
- Vegetables
- Fruit
- Whole grains

Fiber can also be found in some forms of protein such as nuts, seeds and legumes. Best to choose fruits and veggies that are high in fiber.

3. Good fats: are minimally processed fats. They can come from olive oil (such as on a salad), coconut oil in cooking, fat from unsalted raw nuts (especially walnuts), avocados or fish.

4. Pure water: make sure you are drinking enough healthy, pure water. When you consume a lot of fiber from fruits and vegetables, your digestive system requires more water to help the fiber do its job.

Meals, Snacks and the Daily 4 Step Plan

3 Meals and the 4 Step Plan:
Breakfast, Lunch and Dinner

1. Protein: consume 15-20 grams per meal
2. Fiber: consume 8-10 grams per meal from veggies and fruits, some whole grains, or some forms of protein
3. Incorporate good fats
4. Drink pure water

3 Snacks and the 4 Step Plan:
Morning, Afternoon and Evening

1. Protein: consume 8-10 grams per snack
2. Fiber: consume 4-6 grams per snack from veggies and fruits, some whole grains, or some forms of protein
3. Incorporate good fats
4. Drink pure water

The Healthy Food Plate:
A Visual of the Daily 4 Step Plan

Think of the Healthy Food Plate graphic below as a visual image of the Daily 4 Step Plan, in the form of your plate at a meal or snack. The Plate represents an 8 inch dinner plate, or a 6 inch luncheon plate, or a 4 inch snack plate - depending on which meal or snack you are eating. This is an easy way to remember the Daily 4 Step Plan.

The Plate is divided into 4 sections that are not quite even. One section is Healthy Protein and three sections form the Fiber component (Whole Grains + Vegetables + Fruit). The Healthy Fats are a hidden aspect of one or two of the four sections, and the Pure Water is not shown on the plate. Here is the full explanation:

1. **Healthy Protein** – consume 15-20 grams/meal; and 8-10 grams/snack.
- Is important because protein is a necessary building block used throughout your body.
- Should cover a maximum of 25% of the plate.
- Some sources of protein also contain healthy fats (fish, nuts, and seeds).
- Some sources of protein also contain fiber (nuts, seeds and legumes).

2. **Fiber = Whole Grains + Vegetables + Fruits**
- Consume 8-10 grams per meal and 4-6 grams per snack.

- **Whole grains** – are important, but are not absolutely necessary.
    - Are one of the three food categories that contain fiber, as well as vitamins and minerals.
    - Can cover up to a maximum of 25% of the plate, or much less.
    - Important note: if whole grains are omitted, increase the vegetables. (DO NOT substitute highly processed and refined grain products which are high glycemic).

- **Vegetables** – are extremely important.
    - Are the second food category that contains fiber, as well as vitamins, minerals, some protein and antioxidants which your body needs every day.
    - Help to alkalize your body, which is important to maintain a balanced pH level.
    - Should cover a minimum of 30% of the plate.

- **Fruits** – are important but not totally necessary at every meal or snack.
    - Are the third food category that contains fiber, as well as vitamins, minerals and antioxidants– all necessary nutrients for good health.
    - Can cover a maximum of 20% of the plate, or much less.
    - If fruits are omitted – increase the vegetables.

3. **Healthy fats** - a hidden nutrient on the Plate.
   - Are not shown as a category on the Plate because fats are incorporated with the other elements and not consumed individually. For instance – we wouldn't eat a few spoonfuls of olive oil or coconut oil.
   - Could be part of the Healthy Protein (nuts, seeds, fish).
   - Could be added to foods on the Plate in the form of condiments (such as olive oil on a salad) or from cooking (such as light stir-frying of veggies).

4. **Pure Water** – although it is not shown on the plate because it is a beverage, it is still important and needs to be part of the meal.

The bottom line: your food plate should consist of a lot of vegetables and a reasonable amount of protein at every meal. Fruits and whole grains are important too, but not absolutely necessary at every meal, and can be consumed in more limited amounts.

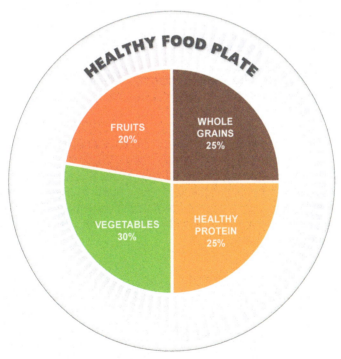

Reasons for Balanced Meals and Snacks

- To keep your blood sugar in the middle or 'performance zone' all day long (not spiking and crashing).

- To keep your metabolism burning evenly

- To give you energy all day long – both mentally and physically

- To give your body the nutrition it needs at intervals throughout the day, which feeds your body's organs and gives you energy.

- To keep you from having very low blood sugar, particularly mid morning and mid afternoon, which creates issues like:
  - brain fog
  - low energy
  - headaches
  - irritability
  - jitters
  - lack of concentration

- To stop impulse eating (grabbing and eating the first food item you see, healthy or not) because you are simply too hungry.

Remember the Sugar Switch Triggers

When you are starting to control your Sugar Switch and shifting from a refined foods lifestyle to a whole foods lifestyle, you need to remember which foods to eliminate permanently, which foods to delete temporarily, and which ones to modify. Here are three reminders:

Reminder #1 – Certain foods to completely eliminate:

As noted in Chapter 3, there are certain food items, your Sugar Switch Triggers, that you need to eliminate while making the transition to a healthier whole foods lifestyle:

- NO sugar
  (use small amounts of stevia, xylitol, berries or fruit instead)
- NO commercial juices
  except limited tomato juice, very limited homemade juices
- NO 0% dairy products or skim milk, NO rice milk beverage
  (our body needs some fat that can come from dairy products; rice milk is high glycemic)
- NO deep fried foods
  very limited pan fried foods with olive oil or coconut oil only
- NO refined junk foods, snacks or fast foods – this includes white rice, refined fast and junk foods, white pastas, baked goods or white wheat flour products. Rule of thumb: if it is a refined fast food it has probably been processed to the point where it has no nutrition in order to make it a fast food.

Reminder #2 – Temporarily remove these foods:

As noted in Chapter 3, temporarily remove these foods while making a transition to a healthier whole foods lifestyle:

- Grains: quinoa, barley, buckwheat, brown rice, whole grain breads
- Potatoes (especially large baking potatoes)
- Dried fruits
- Corn
- Ham
- Beer, wine and other alcoholic beverages

Reminder #3 – Modification of certain foods:

As noted in Chapter 3, modify the consumption of these foods while making a transition to a healthier whole foods lifestyle:

- Homemade juices
- Fried Foods
- Dairy
- Meats

Chapter 6: Protein

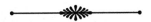

What Is Protein?

Protein: large molecules made up of one or more chains of amino acids

Protein has many functions that affect almost every aspect of our body, such as:

- Helps to form blood cells.
- Plays a role in proper functioning of antibodies to resist infection.
- Are building blocks of body tissue – for maintenance and repair.
- Forms part of our bone structure.
- Is a major component in neurotransmitters, which enable our nerves cells to send and receive messages.
- Replicates DNA.
- Regulates enzymes and hormones.
- Is a catalyst for metabolic reactions within our cells.
- Transports molecules from one location to another in the body.

The amount of protein required depends on age, health status and activity level – the range is from 0.8 grams of protein per kilogram of body weight (for sedentary adults) to 1 gram of protein per kilogram of body weight (for very active or athletic adults).

Note that some groups of people require more, such as athletes, pregnant or breast-feeding women, children, infants, adolescents.

Too much protein can lead to bone loss, kidney disease, high cholesterol and heart problems. Not enough protein in the diet can lead to stunted physical growth, wasting of muscle, anemia and poor brain development.

Animal Protein versus Vegetable Protein

There are pros and cons to each...

Animal protein: from lean red meats, poultry, eggs, fish and seafood, dairy products.
- Has the same overall effect on the body as vegetable protein (does the same job).
- Red meat contains saturated fat.
- Does not contain fiber.

Vegetable protein: from nuts and seeds, beans and legumes, quinoa and buckwheat.
- Has the same overall effect on the body as animal protein (does the same job).
- Does not contain saturated fat.
- Contains fiber.
- Not all vegetable protein sources contain complete protein.

What Is The Best Source of Protein?

There isn't one best source. From my research, I conclude that a well balanced diet with a variety of protein sources is the best way to ensure you are getting enough of all the amino acids your body needs for protein.

Chapter 7: Carbohydrates

What Is a Carbohydrate?

Every carbohydrate (carb) has a sugar molecule as the base, which is made up of a combination of carbon, hydrogen and oxygen. Chains of sugar molecules form starches and fiber.

Our bodies need carbs to have fuel for energy. Basically, the carbs are converted to glucose (blood sugar) and either used immediately or stored in the muscles and the liver, for use later as required.

Types of Carbs

There are three main groups of carbs - sugar, starch and fiber.

1. Sugar – the *simple* form of carbs
    - sugars found naturally in foods such as fruits, vegetables, milk and milk products: these natural sugars from whole foods have nutritional value that our bodies can use in the form of vitamins, minerals, enzymes and phytonutrients.
    - processed sugars that are added to refined foods: these sugars have very little (or no) nutritional value compared to natural sugars from whole foods. Some examples of added processed sugars: brown sugar, corn syrup/sweetener, dextrose, fructose, glucose, high fructose corn syrup (HFCS), invert sugar, maltose, malt sugar, sucrose, sugar, fruit juice concentrates.

2. Starch – a *complex* form of carb
    - consists of sugar units bonded together and can't be used by the body until it is broken down into glucose (through digestion).
    - found in vegetables, whole grains, cooked beans/legumes, peas.

3. Fiber – a *complex* form of carb
    - consists of sugar units bonded together.
    - found in fruits, vegetables, whole grains, peas, cooked beans/legumes, some breads and cereals.
    - the two types of fiber, soluble and insoluble, are both necessary for optimal health.

Not All Carbohydrates Are Healthy

There are **good** carbs and there are **harmful** carbs.

- **Good** carbs are from whole foods, and have nutritional value. Fruits and vegetables, whole grains and legumes all provide carbs that have vitamins, minerals, enzymes and phytonutrients. Some processed grains (breads and cereals) with a very low amount of refining and/or processed sugar could also be nutritious.

- **Harmful** carbs are from highly refined foods that have added processed sugars. These foods contain far less nutrients than whole foods. In fact, many processed foods are completely empty foods, with no nutrition - foods that fill us up, but leave us nutritionally starving.

    These carbs also digest so quickly that they cause the blood sugar to spike, which forces the pancreas to produce large amounts of the fat storing hormone insulin – an issue in many degenerative diseases such as metabolic syndrome, pre-diabetes, diabetes, fatty liver and inflammation.

Good carbohydrates to consume daily:

- Whole foods that contain vitamins, minerals, fiber – all the nutrients that our body can use. These whole foods are mostly low glycemic (unless you eat an excessive amount).

- Fresh fruits – contain fiber, vitamins and minerals: apples, oranges, pears, berries, pineapple, grapefruit, bananas, mangos, kiwi, grapes, pomegranates, lemons, apricots, cherries, peaches, plums, cranberries, rhubarb, dates, and more

- Vegetables - contain great amounts of vitamins, minerals and fiber.
    - Cruciferous vegetables: broccoli, cauliflower, kale, Brussels sprouts, cabbage, bok choy
    - Root vegetables: sweet potato/yam, carrots, beets, Jicama, burdock, parsnips, radish, turnip, rutabaga, onion, ginger
    - Squash – both winter and summer: butternut, acorn, zucchini, spaghetti, hubbard, delicata, kabocha, winter crookneck, turban, yellow crookneck, pumpkin
    - Leafy greens – kale, many kinds of lettuce, spinach, sprouts of all kinds, cilantro, parsley
    - Other nutritious vegetables not mentioned above: avocados, fennel, asparagus

- Healthy grains: quinoa, brown rice (NOT white rice), buckwheat, whole wheat (NOT white processed wheat products), barley

- Beans and legumes, which contain both fiber and protein: kidney beans, chick peas, lentils, black beans, pinto beans, navy beans, fava beans, adzuki beans, black eyed peas, split peas

- Nuts and seeds – most contain fiber, protein and healthy fats: pumpkin seeds, sunflower seeds, sesame seeds, cashews, almonds, brazil nuts, walnuts, pecans

Harmful carbohydrates to AVOID:

- Burgers, hot dogs, fries, onion rings, yam fries and deep fried seafood of any sort...(you get the picture, right?)

- Manufactured "foods" that only look like food, but have absolutely NO nutritional value. Examples are: boxes of whole grain cereals with fruit that do not contain any whole grains or any real fruit, processed cheese slices that are full of dyes, chemicals and artificial flavorings. NOTE: 95% of these manufactured foods are high glycemic.

- Processed foods such as most packaged foods, white rice, white bread and baked goods, pizza, chips, pretzels, any deep fried foods, fast junk foods, candies, cookies, etc.

- Large baking potatoes, including french fries.

- Large amounts of corn (more than about 1/3 cup).

- Sugar (including white sugar, high fructose corn syrup, fructose, maltodextrin, dextrose, and all their derivatives).

- All chemical sweeteners such as sucralose, Splenda, saccharin (aka Sweet'n'Low, Sugar Twin), and aspartame (aka Equal, Nutrasweet, Spoonful).

- Fried foods, including anything breaded.

- Commercial juices.

Chapter 8: Grains

Two Categories of Grains

There are basically two categories for grains: whole grains and processed grains.

NOTE: During the transition from your current refined foods lifestyle to a healthier, low glycemic whole foods lifestyle - ALL grains should be avoided. This is temporary and necessary to keep the blood sugar in the right zone, with no spiking and no crashing.

Once a healthier whole foods lifestyle is achieved, WHOLE grains can be added back into the diet, *with modifications*. Processed grains need to be *permanently deleted* from your whole foods lifestyle.

1. Whole grains – beneficial for health

When grains are minimally processed, they are considered whole grains. They still contain nutritional value for your body and your body is equipped to process them. Essentially, they are exactly the way Mother Nature intended them to be. They contain fiber, vitamins and minerals, which our body can use. Because they contain fiber (and sometimes protein), they are generally lower glycemic. The fiber content slows down the digestive process therefore they don't cause the blood sugar to spike – unless an excessive amount is eaten at one time.

Whole grains include buckwheat, quinoa, brown rice, amaranth, millet, and whole wheat (with the wheat bran and wheat germ intact). Some grains, such as quinoa and buckwheat, also contain protein.

2. **Processed grains – harmful to your health**

Processed grains are refined to the point where they are largely void of nutrition and they are harmful for you. Your body is simply not equipped to handle these empty foods. These processed grains are high glycemic, meaning they digest and turn to blood sugar very quickly, which causes the blood sugar rollercoaster and forces your body to produce excess insulin. These foods are mostly empty calories that fill up your tummy but leave you nutritionally starving. They actually rob you of nutrition and energy because your body has to expend resources and energy to get rid of these toxic refined foods.

Processed grains are found in commercial baked goods including buns, bread, bagels, cakes and cookies, and most commercial cereal products; white pastas; all white flour and flour products including pizza crusts; white rice.

Chapter 9: Fiber

Fiber is another one of the important nutritional factors in balanced eating. Fiber regulates blood sugar by slowing down the digestion process of carbohydrates, so they turn to blood sugar more slowly. This keeps the blood sugar level in the optimal middle zone (not spiking and not crashing).

Fiber plays other important roles in your body as well. It helps the digestive system eliminate waste products through the bowels. It can also lower cholesterol levels. And with fiber rich foods, you can be satisfied between meals, so you are less likely to eat impulsively.

Startling Fiber Facts

Did you know that:

- The typical North American consumes only 15 grams of fiber every day.

- Many medical experts agree that people need to consume from 35-50 grams of fiber a day for optimal health.

- According to several well-controlled studies - people who consume more dietary fiber from foods tend to be less overweight.

- Fiber is linked to the prevention of colon and breast cancer.

- There are two types of fiber: insoluble and soluble. Consuming both types of fiber is important because each of them provide specific benefits.

Soluble Fiber

Soluble fiber dissolves in water. It is found in nuts and seeds, oatmeal, oat bran, most fruits. The benefits of soluble fiber are:

- It lowers total cholesterol and LDL (bad) cholesterol, therefore reducing the risk of heart disease.
- It regulates blood sugar for people with diabetes, metabolic syndrome and helps with weight loss.

Insoluble Fiber

Insoluble fiber does not dissolve in water. It is found in barley, brown rice, whole grain cereals, wheat bran, seeds, and most vegetables. The benefits of insoluble fiber are:

- It removes toxic waste through colon in less time.
- It prevents constipation, hemorrhoids and diverticulosis.
- It helps prevent colon cancer.

IMPORTANT NOTE: There is no need to be too concerned about how much soluble fiber and how much insoluble fiber you are consuming. If you are consuming 35 grams of fiber (or more) per day, it is very likely a good mixture of soluble and insoluble fiber.

Chapter 10: Fats - Good versus Harmful

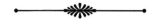

Why Do We Need to Consume Good Fats?

Many of your body's organs (brain and nervous system, heart and circulatory system, skin, hair, and nails) require good fats to keep you healthy and energized every day. Keep in mind that all fats need to be consumed in moderation.

Good Fats

Good Fats include unsaturated fats and coconut oil

1. MUFA's or Monounsaturated fats
MUFA's or Omega 6 fatty acids are from olive oil, peanut oil, avocados, nuts and seeds and other vegetable oils. They are more common in our diet than Omega 3 Fatty Acids, and most people actually get an over-abundance of Omega 6 fatty acids. They can decrease the risk of heart disease because of improved blood cholesterol levels, and can be beneficial in type-2 diabetes by improving insulin levels and blood sugar control.

2. PUFA's or Polyunsaturated fats
PUFA's or Omega 3 fatty acids are building blocks of the brain and nervous system -most people don't get enough Omega 3 fatty acids in their diet. Omega 3 fatty acids come from cold water fish (salmon, mackerel, herring) and from ground flaxseed, flax oil and walnuts. They can decrease the risk of heart disease because of improved blood cholesterol levels, and can be beneficial in type-2 diabetes.

3. Coconut Oil
Coconut oil is controversial, but more and more research tells us it is a good fat. Even though it is a saturated fat (and solid at room temperature), research shows that it is different than saturated fats from animal products. Coconut oil is made up of medium chain fatty acids (MCFAs), which have very different properties than the long chain fatty acids found in animal

saturated fats. MCFAs are healthy for us, and do not cause high cholesterol.

Because of these MCFAs, coconut oil has many benefits – here are just a few:
- It takes less energy and fewer enzymes to digest, thus providing more energy at a quicker rate than other fats.
- It is beneficial in normalizing cholesterol levels, therefore supporting cardiovascular health.
- It reduces our body's need to produce adrenal hormones by normalizing blood sugar levels, increasing energy and reducing stress on our system.
- It increases metabolism, which can help with weight loss.
- It can restore natural saturated fat levels to our cell membranes, and to our skin.
- It is very beneficial for healthy development of children's nervous systems.

Harmful Fats

Harmful Fats include saturated fats and trans fats

1. Unhealthy Saturated Fats

These are mainly from animal sources (fats such as beef fat, pork fat, lard, shortening, and butter). They can increase risk of heart disease by raising total cholesterol levels, particularly LDL (bad) cholesterol and can increase risk of type-2 diabetes. Most saturated fats are solid at room temperature.

2. Very harmful Trans Fats – there are two types

- Synthetic (industrial) trans fats are produced by partial hydrogenation of saturated fats (adding hydrogen to vegetable oil). This is done to increase the shelf life of the fat and make it easier to cook with. These harmful fats are like plastic and virtually never break down!

Synthetic trans fats increase triglycerides (a type of fat found in your blood), which in turn increases the risk of stroke, diabetes, heart attack and heart disease. They increase LDL (bad) cholesterol. They also damage the body's cells by increasing free radicals and causing inflammation.

- Naturally occurring trans fats are found in dairy products and animal sources. They are not as harmful as synthetic trans fats.

Chapter 11: Water

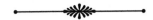

Staying hydrated is very important, since water comprises about 60% of our body weight and almost every system in our body requires water in order to function properly.

Healthy Water is Important

It is important to drink the healthiest water you are able to get. Many municipalities add harmful additives to their tap water, such as fluoride. Ironically, many chemicals are added to municipal water to purify it and those chemicals themselves could be harmful and cause health issues. Most municipal tap water is acid forming in the body, which can cause health issues.

Drinking bottled water does not assure you that it is clean, safe water. Most bottled water is acid forming in the body. Many brands of bottled water are no better than tap water as there are no standards for the quality of bottled water. Bottled water also causes an environmental hazard from the many millions of bottles that are dumped into the landfill sites every year.

Having a good quality water filter on your kitchen sink water supply would be ideal. There are many different kinds on the market, and they are all a little bit different. Best choice would be to have a water filtering system that balances the pH of the water, so the water will not be acid forming.

Health tip: Drinking a glass of room temperature water every morning upon rising is a very good way to get your digestive system going. Squeezing some fresh lemon into the water would be an extra healthy boost.

The Functions of Water

Water performs many functions in our body. Here is a partial list:
- maintains fluid balance
- important for nerve impulses
- transports nutrients and oxygen to our cells
- helps with muscle contraction
- aids digestion and waste removal
- maintains body temperature
- helps dissolve nutrients and minerals so our body can use them
- lubricates our joints
- keeps body tissues moist, such as our mouth, ears and nose

The Benefits of Drinking Enough Healthy Water

There are many benefits of drinking enough water – here are just 7 important benefits:

1. Replacement of natural water loss, which happens through breathing, sweating, normal evaporation through the skin, urination and elimination.
2. Helps to keep our muscles energized (dehydration can cause muscle fatigue).
3. Helps keep our synovial fluids hydrated, which lubricate our joints to keep them healthy.
4. Helps to keep our skin looking great (dehydration can cause the skin to look excessively dry and wrinkly).
5. Helps our kidneys get rid of toxins through urine.
6. Helps our bowels maintain good elimination, especially when our diet contains enough healthy fiber (dehydration can cause constipation).
7. Can help our body lose excess weight: drinking water in place of unhealthy beverages that are full of sugar or chemical sweeteners will help keep our blood sugar balanced and significantly reduce our sugar and/or chemical sweetener intake.

How Much Water Do We Need?

There is no one right answer because there are a number of variables, and we are all unique. Here are the four main variables to consider:

1. How much exercise you are doing, including the type and the duration of exercise (basically more exercise = more sweating and loss of water).

2. What kind of climate you live in, and what altitude (hot and humid climates = more sweating and loss of water).

3. Your health status – some health issues may cause the body to require more water, other health issues may require a reduction in water intake.

4. Women who are pregnant or breastfeeding will require more water to stay hydrated.

Chapter 12: Cravings

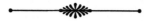

What is a Craving?

The dictionary defines craving as a powerful desire for something. We can all relate to that when it comes to food! Having a craving for something, particularly food, is often considered to be negative, or a sign of weakness (because we feel the need to give in to the craving).

It's definitely true that a craving can actually be caused physically by the food we eat – such as high glycemic food causing the spiking and crashing blood sugar scenario leading to physical cravings. But I believe there could be much more to cravings than that. After all, people who have a low glycemic whole foods lifestyle can still have cravings.

I would like to suggest that there is another side to cravings. Cravings can actually be positive for us. A craving can actually be a sign from our body or from our inner self, telling us that something needs our attention. It could be an outward sign with a hidden inward message. For instance if you are always craving something sweet to eat, is it possible that there is a situation or something in your life that is lacking –like sweetness, joy, love or connectedness?

A craving can have many different meanings, depending upon the person. We are all unique and different. While you might have the same craving as someone else, your craving could have a totally different meaning, message or cause from the other person's craving.

Triggers For Cravings

When you control your Sugar Switch through a healthy whole foods lifestyle, you stop the nasty physical cycle of cravings that causes the rollercoaster of spiking and crashing blood sugar.

When you have a healthy blood sugar level (in that middle zone) all the time, the physical cravings will stop – permanently. There is a caveat though (Isn't there always a caveat?). Veering off your healthy whole foods lifestyle, like being snagged by a season of chocolate and sweets (like Christmas), is enough to get the physical cravings going again. The good news? It is totally reversible!

Nonetheless, we are all human and certain things can indeed start the cravings again. Keep in mind that each person is different, and there isn't just one answer. Each of us have different triggers for cravings – some triggers can be obvious, like high glycemic food, other triggers may actually be hidden and much harder to figure out.

Be a detective! Dig deep.

When you are in detective mode and start analyzing the cravings to figure out what the cause is, it's usually best to start with the most obvious possible culprits. When the obvious culprits have been ruled out, you might need to dig deep and see if there is a hidden message or an important piece of information for you about something that needs your attention.

There are many possible causes. Here is a list, from the obvious to the more hidden:

- Your Sugar Switch has been flipped ON. This can happen from too much refined food, sugar, sweetened beverages or alcohol. It causes your blood sugar to spike and your body to produce excessive amounts of insulin, putting you on that blood sugar rollercoaster of spiking and crashing.

- Consuming artificial sweeteners can be an issue. Chemical artificial sweeteners have been shown to have an effect on a part of our brain. They can actually trick the body into producing excess insulin, even though the blood sugar hasn't physically spiked.

- Your craving could have to do with the seasons. Often we can crave foods that balance the elements of the season. In spring, many people craving detoxifying foods such as citrus foods or leafy greens; in summer it is common to crave cooling foods such as raw foods, salads or ice cream; in the fall we often crave warming and grounding foods like soups, chili and stews.

- Cravings can be caused by hormonal changes in the body. Many women experience this with menstruation, pregnancy or menopause.

- A former craving is suddenly sparked or rekindled by something you saw or by social pressure. Sometimes we see or smell something that brings back a strong memory from our past and we can suddenly find ourselves craving a certain food. One example would be the smell of fresh baked cinnamon buns – the same wonderful aroma you knew when you were growing up, which ignites a desire for that food. Another example is a Christmas gathering where there are many sweets and people are happily indulging in some of your former favorite sugary treats.

- You are thirsty and need to drink some water. Your body could be sending you a message that it needs water and the message could be misunderstood. Try drinking some water, waiting for ten to fifteen minutes, then see if the craving is gone.

- Your body is craving some missing vitamins or minerals. It is possible that your body could be lacking certain vitamins and/or minerals, and it is actually craving nutrition, not sugar. Ramp up your healthy, whole foods lifestyle by increasing the amount of vegetables and fruits you consume. There is some natural sugar in vegetables and fruit, and they are packed with nutrition.

- You might not be getting enough healthy protein and fiber in your daily food intake. If your meals and snacks are not nutritionally balanced, if they don't contain enough fiber or protein, they can leave you unsatisfied. If you skip meals and snacks, you can be hungry between meals. This hunger can easily feel like a craving, or it can lead to low blood sugar where you can have negative effects such as brain fog, headaches, irritability, or feel weak physically. When blood sugar gets low, cravings can happen and grabbing the first available food often happens too, healthy or not.

- Your body could naturally be trying to create balance, which manifests as a craving. Consider the Yin and Yang principles of balance found in traditional Chinese medicine. Yin energy includes raw foods, sugar, alcohol, and even drugs. Yang energy includes animal products, cooked food and materialism. A lifestyle that has an overabundance of yang energy could cause a craving for yin energy to maintain balance. Conversely, an extreme amount of yin energy could cause a craving for yang energy.

- Your craving could be caused by boredom. When we are not busy or when we are bored with what we are doing, our mind can wander and our thoughts can easily move in the direction of cravings.

- You may be experiencing too much stress in your life. You may be feeling completely overwhelmed by what is going on in your life. During times of extreme stress, many people crave comfort food. Most comfort food is highly refined food or junk food.

- Cravings could be a sign that you are seeking comfort or refuge from a particular negative situation or relationship in your life.

- A craving could be an outward sign of an imbalance in your life or lifestyle. Ask yourself if there is something out of balance in your life. Are you craving more love or better relationships in your life? Are you craving more emotional connectedness? Are you craving more joy or pleasure?

- Is there a pattern to your craving? What happened in your life just before the craving started? Does the craving always follow the same scenario in your life?

- Is there something inside you that needs to be expressed? Is there something that is pushed down or suppressed? The craving could be a hidden message of something trying to express itself from inside of you.

- Do you have enough healthy food available when you need it? Planning ahead to make sure you have the right foods in your fridge or cupboard, or the right snacks with you when you are out and about can make a big difference. Sometimes, if we don't have healthy choices within reach, we might start to look for or start to crave previous old favorite foods that are not so healthy. So plan ahead to have healthy choices to fit your schedule, especially for take-along snacks.

- Is it possible that your craving could be part of a self-sabotage syndrome? Sometimes when we are in unfamiliar territory and things are going too well, we crave foods that could throw us off or put us back into familiar territory.

Crowding Out: Fill Your World With Healthy Foods and Beverages:

When you make conscious decisions to fill your world with health food and beverages, you leave no room for unhealthy food and beverages. You are simply too full to fit any more in!

This concept is known as crowding out. You literally crowd out the unhealthy, harmful or negative foods by filling yourself up with an abundance of healthy foods and beverages.

It's a fairly simple concept that takes planning and conscious choice. When you are choosing to eat all healthy foods on a continuous basis, the cravings will most likely just disappear. Your body will be used to the healthy, natural sweetness that is found in fresh fruits and vegetables.

Chapter 13: The Physical Connection

Get Physical!

Exercise and physical movement are necessary for your body to function at an optimal level, including controlling your Sugar Switch. Recent research indicates that having a sedentary lifestyle or sitting at a desk all day long without any physical exercise or movement can be very harmful to your health – possibly even more harmful than smoking!

Huge benefits of Physical Activity

There are so many benefits to exercise! It is amazing how much better the body can function when regular exercise is part of a person's lifestyle. Here is a long list of the benefits of consistent, daily exercise (or at least exercising 3 times per week):

- Controlling your Sugar Switch (blood sugar balancing): Exercise will help regulate your blood sugar, so your body will naturally produce less insulin (that means less of the fat storing hormone).

- More fat burning: Exercise will help your body to produce more glucagon (that means more of the fat burning hormone).

- Internal massage: During exercise your body is moving and your internal organs get a gentle, beneficial massage.

- Metabolic rate: Regular exercise will help build your overall muscle mass, which helps to determine your body's metabolic rate. More muscle mass = higher metabolic rate = more calories being burned, even when you are sleeping. Amazing!

- Digestive health: Regular exercise will help your digestive system by relieving flatulence, and promoting regular elimination. This could also be a factor in avoiding colon cancer.

- Healthy toxin release: Exercise will help promote healthy sweating, releasing toxins through your largest organ, your skin.

- Respiratory and circulatory health: Exercise will help your lungs work at peak level, and help promote good blood circulation. It could also help ease breathing difficulties such as mild asthma.

- Staying young: Studies have shown that increasing your aerobic capacity (increasing the capacity of the heart, lungs and blood vessels) by 15 to 25% could help you look and feel younger, and it could also stimulate new brain cell growth. Your cardiovascular system will benefit, and it could potentially help you live longer.

- Revved up immune system: Regular exercise could help strengthen your immune system, keeping you healthier in the long term.

- Stress relief and help with depression: Regular exercise releases the feel good hormones in the brain (endorphins), which can help release stress and counteract depression.

- Self esteem: Regular exercise has been known to boost a person's confidence and self esteem.

- Physical balance: Regular exercise can help maintain good posture and balance, which are very important for us as we age. Many seniors sustain serious injury from falls due to loss of balance.

- Increased overall energy level: Exercise actually increases a person's physical energy level. It seems counterintuitive because a person has to expend energy to exercise, but in reality it energizes the body.

- Improved sleep: Regular exercise can help you sleep better, resulting in better overall functioning on a daily basis.

- Building bone mass: Targeted exercises and strength training can help build bone mass. This is incredibly important for us as we get older because statistics show that we lose bone mass as we age.

- Exercise benefits women in menopause: According to the Mayo Clinic, there are many benefits of regular exercise for menopausal women. Those benefits include boosting your mood, helping to prevent weight gain, strengthening the bones, reducing the risk of diseases such as heart disease, type-2 diabetes and breast cancer.

- Exercise benefits for men's health: Exercise benefits for men's health includes stress reduction, weight control, and eliminating the risk of heart disease, as well as certain types of cancer. Studies have shown that Kegel exercises can help strengthen a man's pelvic floor muscles. These muscles support the bowel and the bladder and also have an effect on sexual function.

Exercise Does Not Have To Be Boring!

Many people avoid exercising because it is boring and can sometimes be very restrictive. Not all exercise has to be that way. While it is true that certain physical conditions may require specific daily exercises in order to heal properly, general daily physical exercise and movement does not have to be boring and feel like a chore.

Some examples of specific exercises that are required for particular health issues are: strength training exercises (moderate weights) to improve bone density; therapeutic exercises to strengthen muscles after undergoing joint surgery; specific exercises to strengthen the back or neck to keep it healthy.

If you do need to have a therapeutic exercise routine to stay healthy, then find ways to make it fun! Listen to upbeat, motivational music to get you moving! If you need to use a treadmill or elliptical machine – position the machine by a television and watch something that interests you while you get your exercise. If you work out three times per week at a gym, find a buddy to work out with.

Daily exercise can be enjoyable!

Exercise can be as simple and pleasurable as staying active by regularly walking, riding a bicycle on warm summer days, swimming, playing tennis or badminton, playing with your kids or grandkids, playing a game of frisbee with your friends – you get the idea.

Physical movement should be fun! Setting aside the time every day to do something you ENJOY can be good for your mental health. Find a good physical activity that you really adore. Start from your current exercise level, and become more active gradually. Be gentle with yourself, and build up the amount of physical activity you do over a period of weeks or a few months.

Exercise Tips and Ideas

Here are some tips and ideas on how to increase your exercise or daily physical movement:

- Set aside the time by scheduling it into your daily routine - at least 30 minutes every day, and do your best to stick to it! By building it into your daily routine it will become a good habit and won't feel like extra work.

- If you are not used to regular exercise – you will need to start slowly and build up over a period of weeks. Remember: *your present situation is not as important as the direction in which you are moving.* Keep a notebook, have a goal, and write it down. Make note of where you are with exercise today, and formulate a plan to increase your exercise level a little bit each week.

It's not about guilt; it's all about small, manageable steps moving forward. Be gentle with yourself and appreciate yourself for this wonderful journey!

- Walking is a great exercise to start with. If you can, walk outside - the fresh air is very beneficial, mentally and physically. Get a pedometer and measure the number of steps you are taking every day. Start by recording the number of daily steps you take now, and gradually build up the amount of walking you do, having a daily goal in mind such as 10,000 steps. When you reach your goal, start to work on walking faster to help improve your cardiovascular system.

- Walking in winter snow conditions is not always easy due to frigid temperatures and/or ice and snow on the walkways. Perhaps join a fitness facility that has an indoor track or treadmills. Or walk indoors in a shopping mall or in a Plus-15 pedestrian walkway system (such as the one in downtown Calgary).

- Swimming is also a very good exercise, which helps some muscle groups and the cardiovascular system. Aqua exercise classes or swimming lengths are both good options. If you are new to lane swimming (swimming lengths) pace yourself and start out slowly by doing just a few lengths and gradually build up over a period of weeks or months. While lane swimming won't help you lose weight, it will tone many of your muscles – arms, legs and torso, which can keep you slim.

- Join a local gym that holds fitness classes. If fitness classes are really new for you, pace yourself and start out slowly with a beginner class. Gradually increase your workouts with more advanced classes. Gyms have classes such as stationary bicycling (spin class), aerobics classes, and more. Hiring a personal trainer is always an option if you want more targeted exercises and training for a specific reason such as building bone mass by doing strength-training exercises.

Conclusion

There is an unmistakable and vital connection between our daily whole foods lifestyle and our health and wellbeing. Understanding exactly how the food we eat affects us and everything we do is very important. The food we consume on a daily basis makes a very big difference because it feeds us from the cellular level up, and it determines how well our body systems and organs will function.

The Sugar Switch is a key element in the connection between whole foods lifestyle and how well we are. Understanding what The Sugar Switch is all about and how it affects us on a physical level opens the door to learning and to achieving a permanent and healthy whole foods lifestyle that can easily be sustained, every day.

Controlling your Sugar Switch is a matter of making healthy choices. The benefits of controlling your Sugar Switch are nothing short of amazing. You will lose weight without any effort and without more DIETS, you will gain energy, kick the carb/sugar craving permanently, and you will be able to avoid the most common health issues that are prevalent in our society today. These health issues include inflammation, diabetes, obesity, joint pain, fatty liver, low energy, high blood pressure, high cholesterol, high triglycerides and more.

Using the concepts of glycemic index and glycemic load as a guide, avoiding The Sugar Switch triggers, eating a healthy, balanced daily diet and getting physical exercise daily– you will be able to easily maintain ideal body weight and have all the energy you need to do everything you want to do in life!

Being healthy and living a healthy lifestyle is a choice. Making a transition from the standard North American diet to a healthier whole foods lifestyle can be done in small, sustainable steps and it is well worth the effort. Being healthy is a fascinating and wonderful journey!

If you loved the book and want more, please check out my program called Flip The Sugar Switch OFF at:
www.cathyormon.com

Be healthy and live the life of your dreams!

List of Related Information

Glycemic Load and Glycemic Index:

Book - Healthy for Life by Dr. Ray Strand
Dr. Strand's website: www.raystrand.com

David Mendosa is a freelance medical writer specializing in diabetes:
David Mendosa – GI/GL Lists: http://www.mendosa.com/gilists.htm

Online Glycemic Index Database: http://www.gilisting.com/

Harvard Health Publications – GI & GL for 100 Foods: http://www.health.harvard.edu/newsweek/Glycemic_index_and_glycemic_load_for_100_foods.htm

Book – The Blood Sugar Solution by Dr. Mark Hyman
Website: http://www.bloodsugarsolution.com/author/admin/#openModal

Oregon State University – Linus Pauling Institute
http://lpi.oregonstate.edu/infocenter/foods/grains/gigl.html

Insulin Resistance and Metabolic Syndrome:

US National Library of Medicine (PubMed) - Metabolic Syndrome: http://www.ncbi.nlm.nih.gov/pubmedhealth/PMH0004546/

National Diabetes Clearinghouse - Insulin Resistance & Pre-diabetes: http://diabetes.niddk.nih.gov/dm/pubs/insulinresistance/#what

Memory Loss and Alzheimer's Disease:

Dr. Joseph Mercola – High Blood Sugar Levels Linked to Memory Loss
http://articles.mercola.com/sites/articles/archive/2014/12/24/high-blood-sugar-level.aspx

The Mayo Clinic – Diabetes and Alzheimer's Linked
http://www.mayoclinic.org/diseases-conditions/alzheimers-disease/in-depth/diabetes-and-alzheimers/art-20046987

Sugar Consumption and Cancer Risk:

The American Journal of Clinical Nutrition – Sugar and Pancreatic Cancer Risk
http://ajcn.nutrition.org/content/84/5/1171.short

JN The Journal of Nutrition - Insulin, Insulin-Like Growth Factors and Colon Cancer: A Review of the Evidence
http://jn.nutrition.org/content/131/11/3109S.full.pdf+html

Cancer Epidemiology Biomarkers & Prevention – Risk of Colon Cancer
http://cebp.aacrjournals.org/content/6/9/677.short

Hindawi Publishing Corporation – Journal of Diabetes Research - Insulin Resistance and Cancer Risk: An Overview of the Pathogenetic Mechanisms
http://www.hindawi.com/journals/jdr/2012/789174/

About the Author

Cathy Ormon lives in Calgary, Alberta, Canada with her wonderful husband David. She has two incredible grown up children and two fabulous grandchildren, with a third grandchild on the way. Her goal is to help as many people as possible to lose weight, kick the cravings, have more energy, and be healthier – all by controlling their Sugar Switch and harnessing the power of nutrition and whole foods.

My Story – Why I am a Health Coach...

A few short years ago I had a health crisis (crash) and I was unable to obtain guidance from the medical system. That meant I was on my own to find a solution to low energy, joint pain, obesity and systemic inflammation. I was fortunate that synchronistic events took place. Through a friend of a friend, I found a three-month group health coaching program, which I took. That program completely turned my health around! All my life I had been eating the standard North American diet, not realizing how incredibly unhealthy that way of eating really is. The program taught me all about healthy lifestyle, whole foods, the body's insulin production, blood sugar, and how to stop forcing my body to produce excess insulin. It was all about a healthy whole foods lifestyle, and not at all about a diet!

By the end of the three-month health coaching program my weight was well under control, my energy had increased immensely, and the systemic inflammation was totally gone! It was absolutely AMAZING! Within one year I was totally back to good health, including very little joint pain. All of these results came about because of small, sustainable changes in my food intake and my lifestyle choices. This positive experience led me into health coaching. I am passionate about helping others to lose weight *without dieting*, to kick the sugar and carb cravings, to increase their energy and to be the healthiest they can be – and at the same time avoid or even reverse common chronic health issues.

Learning about what I now call The Sugar Switch and how to control it was a very powerful game changer for me! It has been such an important and powerful change for me that I have been inspired to write this book, and a corresponding health coaching program. I am happy to help others who may be experiencing relentless sugar cravings, weight issues, low energy issues, joint pain and possibly other signs of inflammation.

If this book ignites a spark in you to take action and you would like more information please visit my website at **www.cathyormon.com** or contact me at **cathy@cathyormon.com**

My sincere hope is that this book and the information it contains will be a powerful and very positive game changer for you!

To your good health,

Cathy Ormon, CHC, AADP
The Sugar Switch Guru

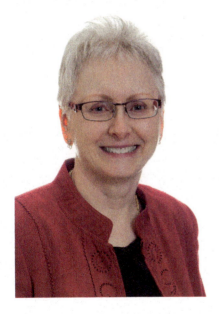